# 30 Day Whole Food Challenge

The Complete 30 Day Whole Food Challenge to Lose Weight and Live a Healthier Lifestyle

D1259068

**BY: Sarah Stewart**

# Table of Content      **Page**

# Chapter 1- SO, JUST WHAT ARE WHOLE FOODS?

You may have heard the term whole foods before and wondered what exactly that means. Simply put, whole foods are foods you eat in their natural state. If a food is something you could grow or hunt, then you are on the right track. This means meat, poultry, and chicken are all green lights. Eggs are good too! On a whole food diet or challenge, you can eat as many vegetables as you want. Fruits are good in moderation and fats that come from healthy sources such as oils and seeds. Fresh herbs, garlic, and most dried herbs are fine to consume as well.

## OK, THEN WHAT IS OFF-LIMITS?

You may think it seems like there are many of your favorite foods on the "Do Not Eat List" but the rewards you will reap for following this plan for 30 consecutive days or longer far outweigh giving anything up. Basically, no junk food, processed foods, pre-packaged foods etc. Sugar is off-limits, real or artificial. This does include alcohol. For thirty days, you need to cut out dairy, grains, legumes (beans, lentils, soy). Not just soy beans but soy sauce as well. Dairy includes milk, yogurt, ice-cream, Greek yogurt and any other type of animal milk products. MSG, a food additive is also forbidden.

## NOW, WHY WOULD I WANT TO DO THIS?

Well, I am glad you asked! The benefits of doing a whole food diet for 30 days far outweigh the loss of your favorite foods. Certain foods could be causing your lack of energy, your low libido or your joint inflammation. Doing the 30-day whole food diet "resets" your body and gives you the ability to add foods in one at a time. Some people find though that once the banned foods are eliminated they no longer desire to consume them. On this diet, you will find your skin looks better, you have more energy, you have less pain and generally you just feel better. You may find that you get headaches less frequently and your allergies clear up. Not to mention the best part! You will lose weight. Who doesn't love that?

"Take time to deliberate, but when the time for action has arrived, stop thinking and go in."
~Napolean Bonaparte

# WHAT AILMENTS WILL THIS HELP?

The Whole Food Challenge can help clear up or improve a myriad of medical conditions. The majority of users who succeed in sticking it out for a month often stay on the diet, at least for the most part, because of the astounding changes they experience.

This diet can help with...

- Fibromyalgia
- High Cholesterol
- High Blood Pressure
- Heartburn
- Celiac Disease
- Allergies
- Migraines
- Poly Cystic Ovarian Disease
- Celiac Disease
- Diverticulitis
- Skin Conditions, including hives
- Allergies
- Asthma
- IBS

- Crohn's Disease
- Chronic Pain- especially in your joints
  Exhaustion -You may feel even more tired
  the first several days, it happened to me so
  do not give up because after the first several
  days you will have a marked increase in
  energy.
  "Health is a state of complete physical,
  mental and social well-being, and not merely
  the absence of disease or infirmity." ~World
  Health Organization

## WON'T IT BE HARD?

When starting this diet, most people want to know how hard it will be. The level of difficulty really depends on how much you use the banned foods currently. Sugar can be addictive and if you are drinking a lot of soda every day then your body has learned to crave the sugar. We will break this addiction! The first week will be the hardest and then it will get easier but remember it is just thirty days. I imagine you have done more difficult things in your life. Have you ever studied for exams? Locked yourself out of the house? Spent a week on vacation with your in-laws? See, there are harder things than eating healthy for a month and I have faith in you!

"Don't dwell on what went wrong. Instead, focus on what to do next. Spend your energies on moving forward toward finding the answer." ~Denis Waitley

"You are braver than you believe, stronger than you seem, and smarter than you think." ~Christopher Robin

## WHAT IF I MESS UP?

"There are only two options regarding commitment; you're either in or you're out. There's no such thing as life in-between." ~Pat Riley

"Don't dwell on what went wrong. Instead, focus on what to do next. Spend your energies on moving forward toward finding the answer." ~Denis Waitley

# Chapter 2-HOW DO I BEGIN?

The first thing to do is get rid of anything that is not on the approved foods list. Donate the food to a food bank. Be vigilant and make sure you get everything out. Get the whole family on it. It is just a month, right? Even kids can benefit greatly from this challenge. If you do not have a lot of Tupperware, then pick some up. Having snacks will help you through the month and the best way to do that is to have fruits and veggies ready to snack on. If you cut them up as soon as you get home from the market, then they are just as easy to grab a bag of chips used to be. Having a water bottle is smart because drinking water consistently not only keeps you feeling full but is immensely good for your body. The last thing to do is get a notebook to plan your meals. This will save you time and frustration.

## HOW CAN I GET THE WHOLE FAMILY INVOLVED?

If you are living with a family, then you may be wondering how you will take the Whole Foods Challenge for 30 days and still make your family whatever they want for dinner. I would encourage you not to even think about that. Get the whole family in on it! Kids too! It is just 30 days, remember? Your kids will be just fine without sugar for 30 days and will honestly be better off without it. Getting kids involved can seem daunting but one way that almost always works is offering a prize. Kids thrive on competition, especially the friendly kind! So, offer some rewards or prizes based on certain behaviors or goals. It will not be hard to get your kids excited about something like this when they know they can go to a movie at the theater or pick out a new toy when the 30 days are up. Now, obviously, I am not suggesting that anyone make a habit out of rewarding kids to eat healthily. You are the parent and you dictate what they eat. However, this reward will make the challenge that much more fun for them and at the end of the 30 days they will have discovered new foods they enjoy and gotten rid of those nasty sugar cravings. That is a great reward for you! Living healthy is a lifestyle, not just a challenge, and the whole family can reap the life-changing, lifesaving rewards in the end.

# SHOULD I HAVE A CHALLENGE BUDDY?

Well, sure! Having a buddy to go through the 30 Day Whole Food Challenge is a great idea! Of course, I know you can do it on your own. I have faith in you! However, having someone to be accountable to can make a huge difference. Cheating on this challenge is not allowed and if you have no one to be accountable to then you may find it easier to cheat. When you are working together you find yourself sticking through the hard days just so you can tell your partner that you made it through another day! Plus, having someone go through the challenge with you means that you have someone to share your ups and downs with and they will understand exactly how you feel! Check in with each other once a day even if it is just a text message.

If you are doing the challenge without a buddy, then tell your friends and family! They will be happy for you and support you and you will be glad to have their encouragement. Who knows! You may just encourage them to jump head first into the challenge too!

"Whenever you do a thing, act as if all the world were watching." ~Thomas Jefferson

## WHAT ABOUT NAYSAYERS?

There will always be naysayers in life and when it comes to doing the 30 day whole foods challenge you may hear something negative. This may not be outright negativity and the person may still be proud of you for doing the diet but you may still encounter these situations.

Jealousy- When someone is jealous they often feel resentful of your success. It may be hard for them to celebrate your successes while they are feeling bad about their own failures. Try not to get upset! Maybe invite them to do it with you? Encourage them on their own journey and if the negativity continues then just stop talking health and diet with that person and focus on something you can both enjoy together happily.

"Just this one time-ers"- It is important on the 30-day challenge to stick to the plan and not cheat, even once, because then you have to start over. Anytime you are following a lifestyle change and decide to give up something such as sugars, bread or caffeine. That is your choice and if you don't ever want to break it then good for you! No one should tell you otherwise but the truth of the situation is that some people will try to tell you otherwise and may even get upset when you will not break your diet and stick to your willpower. This is going to happen at birthday parties. "Come on, it's a party, you can't have one piece of cake?" This is going to happen at work. "We are going out for cocktails. Don't you want to be part of the team?" It might happen at your mom's. "But I spent all day making your favorite chocolate cake and you won't even try it?" Just smile and say "No thank you, it is a choice I have made for my health. I hope you understand."

If they do not that is there hang-up and you cannot let someone else's hang ups get in the way of your life choices. It is your body! You only get one! So, if you want to skip cocktails after work so be it!

"Whatever course you decide upon, there is always someone to tell you that you are wrong. There are always difficulties arising which tempt you to believe that your critics are right. To map out a course of action and follow it to an end requires courage."
~Ralph Waldo Emerson

"People may doubt what you say, but they will believe what you do." ~Lewis Cass

# HOW CAN I STAY MOTIVATED?

"Motivation is what gets you started. Habit is what keeps you going." ~Jim Rohn

One day at a time! Motivation comes in many forms. Why are you wanting to do this challenge? Do you have health problems, weight issues or simply a desire to live a healthier life? That is what will get you started! How great you feel as the challenge goes on is what will keep you motivated!

They say it takes 21 days for an action to become a habit. Now, I don't know who "they" are but "they" are right! I can attest to that personally. This challenge may seem a bit overwhelming at first, depending on where you are at when you begin, but it will get better.

By the end of the challenge meal planning, food prep and eating healthy and whole will become second nature. How great is that?

One thing that can really help are reminders of what you want to do. Hang up pictures of the size you want to get to, a hike you want to complete or different things you want to do when you are healthier. Hang them all over the house. Hang them on the fridge and the pantry and use them as a visual reminder of what you are accomplishing and everything you are gaining from this experience.

"You have to have confidence in your ability, and then be tough enough to follow through." ~Rosalynn Carter

## QUOTES AND MANTRAS TO KEEP YOU GOING

I CAN DO THIS! I AM WORTH IT! I WILL SUCCEED!

WHOLE FOODS=WHOLE LIFE=WHOLE ME

I AM RESETTING MY BODY AND MY BODY IS BEAUTIFUL!

I AM WORTHY OF A HEALTHY LIFESTYLE.

I CAN DO ANYTHING FOR 30 DAYS.

"Great things are not done by impulse, but by a series of small things brought together." ~Vincent Van Gogh

"You will never change your life until you change something you do daily." ~Mike Murdock

"Habit is habit and not to be flung out of the window by any man, but coaxed downstairs a step at a time." ~Mark Twain

"It's not who you think you are that holds you back; it's who you think you're not." ~Unknown

"First thing every morning before you arise, say out loud, 'I believe', three times." ~Norman Vincent Peale

"Don't wait until everything is just right. It will never be perfect. There will always be challenges, obstacles and less than perfect conditions. So what. Get started now. With each step you take, you will grow stronger and stronger, more and more skilled, more and more self-confident and more and more successful." ~Mark Victor Hansen

"No matter who you are, no matter what you do, you absolutely, positively do have the power to change." ~Bill Phillips

"What would you attempt to do if you knew you could not fail?" ~Dr. Robert Schuller

"Put all excuses aside and remember this: YOU are capable." ~Zig Ziglar

"Never let the fear of striking out get in your way." ~George Herman "Babe" Ruth

"Act as if everything you do makes a difference. It does." ~William James

"Where you start is not as important as where you finish." ~Zig Ziglar

"You have to have the bad days to appreciate the good ones." ~Unknown

"In order to change we must be sick and tired of being sick and tired." ~Unknown

"Twenty years from now, you'll be more disappointed by the things you didn't do, than the ones you did." ~Mark Twain

"If I am not good to myself, how can I expect anyone else to be?" ~Maya Angelou

# Chapter 3- APPROVED FOODS LIST

I have done my best to list every option but any fruits and vegetables are okay. (if they are not fried) There are no sneaking French fries in on this diet! One thing you need to remember is that you must stick with this for the whole thirty days. Cheating on the diet is cheating you because your body will not get the affects you desire. If you slip up or you sneak something, then basically the process stops and you have to begin again. Be vigilant over the thirty days and I promise you by the end you will feel like a new person!

"Processed foods not only extend the shelf life, but they extend the waistline as well." ~Karen Sessions

"Don't eat anything your great-great grandmother wouldn't recognize as food." ~Michael Pollan

## GHEE- WHAT THE HECK IS GHEE?

You will notice on your "Oils and Other" list that ghee is listed. You may be wondering what the heck is ghee? Well, to put it simply ghee is a type of liquid clarified butter. When the butter is clarified, it is devoid of milk proteins that do not mesh up well with this diet and can get in the way of your success. It is commonly made from cows and buffalo. You can occasionally use this substance in your meals as a butter substitute but do not use it often as you are trying to learn how to eat whole foods only. You can find it online or in some grocery stores.

# FRUIT

- Strawberries
- Blueberries
- Raspberries
- Blackberries
- Grapes
- Bananas
- Grapefruit
- Oranges
- Cantaloupe
- Watermelon
- Honeydew Melon
- Papaya
- Mango
- Prickly Pear
- Star Fruit
- Pineapple
- Tangerine
- Ugli Fruit
- Kiwi
- Kumquat
- Nectarine
- Paw Paw

- Fig
- Persimmon
- Applesauce- make sure no sugar is added
- Apricots
- Pear

# VEGETABLES

- Iceberg Lettuce
- Romaine Lettuce
- Green Beans
- Corn
- Okra
- Broccoli
- Cauliflower
- Carrots
- Celery
- Peppers
- Romaine Lettuce
- Kale
- Spinach
- Asparagus
- Red Potatoes
- White Potatoes
- Sweet Potatoes
- Cabbage
- Zucchini
- Cucumber
- Squash
- Pumpkin

- Tomato
- Onion
- Mushrooms
- Broccolini
- Peas
- Brussel Sprouts
- Artichoke
- Parsnip
- Canned Crushed Tomatoes or paste is acceptable as long as there is nothing added to the tomatoes
- Avocado

## MEAT

Lunch meat and sausage (unless you make your own approved sausage) are not allowed they are processed but canned meat is okay only if the only ingredient listed is the meat itself. Lean cuts of beef are the best, stay away from fatty meats. Fish is always a smart choice.

- Chicken
- Turkey
- Cornish Hens
- Quail
- Duck
- Beef
- Pork
- Venison
- Bison
- Salmon
- Shrimp
- Crab
- Snapper
- Cod
- Trout
- Bass

- Perch
- Tuna
- Mahi Mahi
- Lobster
- Swordfish
- Scallops
- Clams
- Walleye
- Catfish

## FRESH HERBS

Fresh herbs are going to be a lifesaver to add flavor to your dishes! You can use dried herbs as well. If you are using a seasoning mix, then you need to carefully check the ingredient label to ensure it does not contain sugar or any unhealthy additives.

- Chives
- Garlic
- Oregano
- Parsley
- Mint
- Cinnamon
- Basil
- Sage
- Thyme
- Lemongrass
- Ginger
- Cumin
- Paprika
- Salt
- Pepper
- Red pepper
- Chilies

- Cloves
- Nutmeg
- Bay Leaf
- Ground Mustard
- Rosemary
- Cayenne Pepper

# NUTS AND SEEDS

- Walnuts
- Pine Nuts
- Pistachios
- Macadamia Nuts
- Almonds
- Sunflower Seeds
- Pumpkin Seeds

## OILS AND OTHER

- Olive Oil- Extra Virgin is best for making dressings or drizzling on meals
- Coconut Oil- unrefined
- Sesame Oil- occasionally only
- Balsamic Vinegar
- Rice Vinegar
- White Vinegar
- Red Wine Vinegar

Malt vinegar, like the kind you would put on French fries at a sub shop, is not allowed.

- Cocoa- make sure it is 100% cocoa.
- Hot sauce- check ingredient label, no added sugar or MSG.
- Pickles-no sugar or MSG added-pickle chips make a great snack!
- Relish-no sugar or MSG added
- Capers-no sugar or MSG added
- Curry Paste- green, red and yellow are all allowed
- Almond Flour
- Fish sauce, check for no added sugars

- Beef broth- cannot have any added sugar or MSG
- Chicken broth- cannot have any added sugar or MSG
- Ghee-occasionally only

## IS THERE ANYTHING I CAN BUY AT THE STORE?

Yes, and thank you for asking! There are some things you can buy at the store to help you on your 30 day whole foods challenge and healthier lifestyle. Check out some of these three choices while you are on your 30 day challenge.

1.  Spices- Check out Primal Palate. You can find them at www.primalpalate.com. They have a huge selection of spices as well as an amazing recipe collection that filters for all sorts of dietary restrictions or concerns. Most spices you buy at the grocery store are okay but avoid the mixed blends a lot of them add sugar. You do not want to see anything in the ingredients label except for the spice itself.

2.  Bacon- Generally choosing bacon that is cured with salt and not sugar is good for this challenge. You do want to avoid anything that is flavored. If you are looking for a bacon that is also free of nitrates, then check out Naked Bacon! You can find them at www.nakedbaconco.com. Bonus! They also

make sausage that you can eat as well!

Oooh! Breakfast just got more exciting!

3. Bison- Have you ever had bison meat? It is truly delicious and it is healthy! One brand that offers bison meat that will work on this challenge is Honest Bison. Not to be confused with their competition "the Lying Bison"! You can check out their website at www.thehonestbison.com.

4.

# Chapter 4- WHAT VITAMINS WILL I GET ON THIS PLAN?

The vitamins you get on this diet will depend on which foods you are eating. Let's take a look at some of the main foods and what nutrients they offer you. It is important that you incorporate a variety of foods into your diet to ensure that you are getting all of the different nutrients you need in a wholesome, well-rounded diet.

1. Apples- Apples are known to be high in both fiber and Vitamin C. The skin is one of the healthiest parts so make sure that you eat that part too!

2. Apricots- Apricots are simply delicious! They are little but full of flavor. Apricots have dietary fiber, potassium and copper. They can also give you a nice boost of Vitamin C!

3. Blueberries- Blueberries pack a powerful antioxidant punch and a dose of vitamin K. They should be eaten raw to get the most benefits.

4. Bananas- Bananas offer good amounts of potassium and vitamin B6. They are an easy to grab snack for when you are on the go!

5. Broccoli- Broccoli is a great source for vitamins K and C as well as folate and fiber. Also, broccoli is known to help with inflammation.

6. Beef- Lean beef is something you will enjoy a couple days a week on your challenge. Protein is key when it comes to beef because beef is chock full of protein! It also offers up Zinc and vitamin B6 as well.

7. Chicken- Chicken is one of the most versatile foods available. You can cook it in so many ways and so many flavors it is hard to get bored of it! It is high in protein and vitamin B6.

8. Corn- Corn! I love corn! It is so sweet and delicious! Add a little salt, skip the butter, and you have a delicious side dish. Boiled or grilled, frozen or fresh, all corn is delicious. Corn is another versatile vegetable that can go just about anywhere. Corn is full of phosphorus, dietary fiber and pantothenic

acid. Corn also boats the added benefit of Vitamin B6.

9. Cabbage- Cabbage is one of those foods you probably do not think about very often. It is crunchy though and makes a great addition to any salad. It is full of fiber, Vitamins C, K and B6 plus manganese and folate.

10. Carrots- Carrots are a nice crunchy snack that you can eat both raw and cooked. They are chock full of vitamins such as B6, B1, C, E and B2. Carrots are also a great source of biotin, dietary fiber and potassium.

11. Eggs- Eggs are a lifesaver on the Whole Foods challenge! You can add just about anything to an egg and there are so many ways to cook it. Eggs offer you amino acids as well as choline and selenium. Eggs also give you protein and vitamins B12 and D.

12. Fish- If you aren't a fish lover yet then now is the perfect time to give it a try. Fish makes dips and patties. Fish is good over salads or cooked on a grill. Fish is chock full of protein and vitamin D.

13. Figs- Figs are an often-overlooked fruit. Most people only eat then in a Newton! However, they are pretty delicious and good for you! They deliver fiber, magnesium, calcium and potassium.

14. Grapes- Yum! Grapes are the perfect poppable snack! They contain resveratrol, beta-carotene and vitamin K.

15. Green Beans- Green Beans! Oh, green beans! You are so healthy for me! Green beans are full of things that are good for you. Green beans boast copper, phosphorus, calcium, magnesium, potassium and protein. They also offer Vitamins B1, B6 and Vitamin E.

16. Kale- Holy Beta-Carotene! Holy vitamin K! Holy Vitamin C! One serving of kale has got you covered with all three of the above nutrients.  Stick some in your daily salad!

17. Kiwi- Kiwi is a fruit that you either love or hate. Usually, you will find it in a fruit salad. It is full of dietary fiber and potassium as well as folate and copper. It offers up Vitamins C,

K and E. So pick one up today and see if you love it!

18.  Lobster- If you are lucky enough to eat lobster you are lucky enough! If you are a fan of lobster, you understand. Lobster has Vitamin B12, phosphorus, zinc and protein. It is high in sodium though so if you are

avoiding salt skip the lobster. If you need more salt, well then, consider yourself lucky!

19. Mangoes- Mangoes are a sweet, tropical fruit and a great choice for dessert. Mangoes are high in sugar so they are a once and a while fruit treat. They are full of vitamins A, C and B6.

20. Onions- Onions are my very favorite vegetable! I simply love them, cooked or raw! You can get white onions, yellow onions, red onions and candy onions depending on what you are using them for. They have Vitamins B1, B6 and C. They also offer up folate, dietary fiber and potassium.

21. Pineapple- Pineapple, fresh pineapple is absolutely delicious! It is sweet and

refreshing and a great way to have a sweet treat. Pineapple is chock full of pantothenic acid, dietary fiber, folate and copper plus an array of vitamins. Pineapple offers up Vitamins B1, B6 and C.

22. Macadamia Nuts- Macadamia nuts may be expensive but they are delicious and good for you too! They give you lots of minerals including magnesium, calcium, iron and zinc. They also have a little vitamin B1. They are good on their own or thrown in a fruit salad!

23. Plum- Plums are not only beautiful shades of purple but immensely satisfying and delicious! Plums boast the nutrients potassium and vitamins C and K. They are also a good source of fiber.

24. Spinach- Popeye was on to something! Spinach does make our bodies healthy and strong! Zinc, Potassium, Folate, Calcium plus vitamins B2, B6, E and C just to name a few! Spinach is delicious both raw and cooked and baby spinach makes a great bed of greens for vegetables and meat.

25. Squash- Squash is another one of those versatile vegetables that people can use for many different types of dishes. Squash is a great source for protein, folate and magnesium. Squash also contains dietary fiber and Vitamin C.

26. Tomato- Tomatoes are one of the most versatile fruits. Fruit? Yes, even though I put it on the veggie list, tomatoes are actually a fruit. You can eat them raw or cooked. You can slice them, dice them, stew them sauce them. Tomatoes are a great source of the antioxidant lypocene, as well as the vitamins A, C, K and B6. Tomatoes also boast the nutrients folate, potassium, magnesium and fiber.

27. Zucchini- Zucchini is an underappreciated food but you should give it a shot! It is good both raw and cooked. I prefer it cooked! It has dietary fiber, protein, folate and potassium. Plus, it offers Vitamin C! You can even make "noodles" out of zucchini. They are called zoodles! Doesn't that just make you want to smile?

# Chapter 5- WAIT! I HAVE MORE QUESTIONS! LIKE, WHAT IS MSG?

According to, the Mayo Clinic, MSG is "Monosodium glutamate (MSG) is a flavor enhancer commonly added to Chinese food, canned vegetables, soups and processed meats. The Food and Drug Administration (FDA) has classified MSG as a food ingredient that's "generally recognized as safe," but its use remains controversial."

In layman's terms, this "flavor enhancer" tricks your brain into craving these types of foods. Honestly, it is often used just to get you to buy processed foods more and more. We are on to them now, though, aren't we? The tricky part is that MSG goes by a plethora of names and can be easy to miss. On this diet, if you do not recognize and ingredient you should probably skip the item. Just in case, though, here is a comprehensive list of names for MSG or its friends. I got this list from www.hungryforchange.tv.

➢ Glutamic Acid (E 620)2
➢ Glutamate (E 620)
➢ Monosodium Glutamate (E 621)

- Monopotassium Glutamate (E 622)
- Calcium Glutamate (E 623)
- Monoammonium Glutamate (E 624)
- Magnesium Glutamate (E 625)
- Natrium Glutamate
- Yeast Extract
- Anything hydrolyzed
- Any hydrolyzed protein
- Calcium Caseinate
- Sodium Caseinate
- Yeast Food
- Yeast Nutrient
- Autolyzed Yeast
- Gelatin
- Textured Protein
- Soy Protein Isolate
- Whey Protein Isolate
- Anything: protein
- Vetsin
- Ajinomoto
- Carrageenan (E 407)
- Bouillon and broth
- Stock
- Any flavors or flavoring

- Maltodextrin
- Citric acid, Citrate (E 330)
- Anything ultra-pasteurized
- Barley malt
- Pectin (E 440)
- Protease
- Anything enzyme modified
- Anything containing enzymes
- Malt extract
- Soy sauce
- Soy sauce extract
- Anything protein fortified
- Seasonings

MSG can actually make people very ill. For years my husband would get sick at different restaurants and we could not figure out the rhyme or reason. So, we started asking about MSG. Avoiding it at all costs has made a huge difference in how he feels after eating. So, speak up! If you are planning to go out to eat, on or after this challenge, ask the staff about MSG and avoid it at all costs. Let your taste buds learn to crave natural whole foods and not the processed junk.

## CAN I BAKE?

The honest truth is no. You may be looking at the ingredients thinking hmm... almond flour? Cocoa? Eggs? I bet I can make a cake out of that. Maybe you could. However, you are learning to eat these foods as whole foods. Putting them together is not quite the same thing. Plus you are trying to retrain your brain. That means learning to live without the sweet stuff. Learning to be okay without pies, cookies, cakes, brownies and candy. Learning that saying no to a sweet treat is not depriving yourself but empowering yourself to be a healthier version of you! As the sugar leaves your body, as chemicals like MSG leave your body you will notice that the whole foods taste so much better. A piece of fruit for dessert will be all of the sweetness your body craves. How awesome will that be? That is not to say you will never have a piece of birthday cake again but when you do it will be a treat. One you don't want on a regular basis. You have the power and you CAN do this!

## SHOULD I EXERCISE?

First things first, I am not a doctor. I am not qualified to give you medical advice. So, if you are not currently exercising then please check with a doctor before you start an exercise program.

That being said, let's assume you have spoken to your doctor and got the green light, now I can answer your question. Should you exercise? Why not?

The first few days on this diet are going to be tiring. You will feel fatigued and exhausted but then after your body adjusts to the new menu you will feel more energetic and have less joint pain.

Start with walking! Walking is easy on the joints, you can do it anywhere and anyone can join in. Try and get the whole family out on a nice walk every day or so. After you are used to walking then do not be afraid to branch out. Perhaps, try a higher impact aerobic workout and begin strength training. Look into yoga or Pilates and see which one you like!

Try different activities and mix it up! Enjoy the process of becoming more active and feeling great!

"Those who think they have not time for bodily exercise will sooner or later have to find time for illness." ~Edward Stanley

"Too many people confine their exercise to jumping to conclusions, running up bills, stretching the truth, bending over backwards, lying down on the job, sidestepping responsibility and pushing their luck." ~Anonymous

"Movement is a medicine for creating change in a person's physical, emotional, and mental states." ~Carol Welch

"Walking is the best possible exercise. Habituate yourself to walk very far." ~Thomas Jefferson

# WHAT ABOUT THE SCALE?

Stay away from that scale. You are doing this for your health, weight loss may be a great motivation, however, your health should be the main focus. So, focus on changing your eating habits.

Weight can fluctuate daily, sometimes hourly, and you do not want the scale to influence or hinder your ability to stick it out for the entire 30 day challenge.

If you have to give your scale to the neighbor to hide! Believe me, it will be a nice break to not look at it every day and when day 30 rolls around you will be pleasantly surprised to see what the scale says.

For someone who has been eating a diet full of sugars and processed foods there is a good chance you will see a drastic change! Keep eating healthy and keep exercising if you want to keep the weight off for good.

# WON'T I GET BORED OF SALAD?

It is easy to assume that you will get bored of salad and honestly if you have been eating a lot of french fries and chicken nuggets for lunch every day this is going to be a change. However, the key to not getting bored of salad is mixing it up! Your taste buds will adjust and your palette will begin to discern between all of the different tastes and textures of the various vegetables, oils, nuts and meats. There are literally thousands of different combinations when it comes to making a salad.

Spinach and kale are very healthy and you may be thinking "Ew! What is wrong with this lady!" but baby spinach and baby kale are much less bitter and still pack a powerful punch of nutrients. Spices will be your friend, as will all the different types of oils and vinegar that allow you to mix and match different tastes with different veggies and meats.

# HOW TO DRINK MORE WATER

Drinking water is an important part of a healthy lifestyle and that truth does not change as you embark on the 30 day whole foods challenge. Drinking 8-10 glasses of water a day is your goal.

Being properly hydrated will help you to feel full throughout the day, keep your skin looking soft and beautiful and aide in weight loss and digestion.

One way that I have found, that works in our household, is to get a water cooler. You can have water delivered or you can go get refills at your local grocery store every month. We each have our own water bottle, I bought the nice insulated kind since I wanted them to last, and we fill them up as needed. I have found that my kids drink a lot more water than they did before this.

Even if you do not get a water cooler it is still smart to use the water bottles. That way you can carry it with you and always have water on hand. Before long sipping water all day long will become second nature and you will be better off for it!

# Chapter 6- IS MEAL PLANNING HARD?

Meal Planning is not hard. What it can be is time-consuming. Especially if you are on a processed foods diet now and the only whole food you can think of is salad and grilled chicken. It takes practice and re-training your brain to get used to creating whole food meal plans. Once you get used to it meal planning will feel like a breeze. It is always the first several days that are going to be the hardest. Look over the approved food lists. Copy and paste them into a Word Doc and print them out. This can be a great starting point for a supermarket list. Make a pact with yourself to try one new food a day. Take the time to think out your meal plan and grocery shop for all of your ingredients. It is much easier to cheat when you have had a long day and you can't decide what to eat. If you have the ingredients prepped and ready to go and you know exactly what you are making, then you are much more likely to succeed. Bring prepared in this challenge is definitely of great benefit and will help you succeed.

## HOW DO I COMPLETE WEEKLY PREP

First things first, if you do not have any Tupperware or plastic containers then now is the time to invest. Having your fruits and veggies washed chopped and ready to go is immensely helpful and makes snacking a breeze. However, you do need something to put them in. Ziploc bags can work well too. After you have planned your meals it is important that you get to chopping. Chop up all your fruits and veggies for 3 days at a time, so maybe Sundays and Wednesdays you would do it. Choose two days that work with your personal schedule. Make sure you chop up carrots, celery and cucumbers for easy to grab snacks. Wash your grapes, slice your strawberries and cut your cantaloupe. This is especially helpful if you are cooking for a family or trying to encourage your family to eat healthier. When kids (and adults) have easy access to healthy foods, the way chips and cookies used to be accessible, then they are more likely to grab them. If you make a tuna salad recipe make enough for two meals. Cook up some meat, slice it up and have it ready to add to salads. Roast some nuts or seeds and place them in Ziploc bags to grab for snacks throughout the week. The key to sticking to this challenge without feeling overwhelmed is kitchen prep. Twice a week is all you need to ensure the next 3-4 days go off without a hitch.

# WHAT IS A PROPER PORTION SIZE?

If you have struggled with overeating in your life one of the things you may have struggled with is portion control. Portion control can seem daunting. Who has time to cut and measure and weight everything they eat? I hear you, it can be time consuming. The good thing is that eventually if you follow these tips and tricks you will begin to start having the ability to eyeball your food and get the right portion regardless of whether you weigh it. It does not hurt though, if you are able, to pick up a food scale and start this journey off on the right foot. For the times, though that you are not able to weight your food here is a handy cheat guide!

Protein- protein is one of the most important foods on this challenge, especially since it will help you to feel energized and satisfied, which makes sticking to the diet that much easier. A serving of meat is going to be about the size of a deck of cards. You should be eating meat or fish 2-3 times a day. Protein also includes your nuts. Nuts are a great energizing snack that are packed full of goodness for you! A serving of nuts is about the size of a ping pong ball! A serving of nuts several times a week is a great way to sneak protein into your diet.

Grains- For this challenge grains are on your "no-no" list. Since I want you to move forward after this challenge with all the tools you need to succeed, and some of you are going to eat bread again, I am including the portion sizes for grains as well. When you are thinking of cooked grains think about the size of a tennis ball. If you are like me the amount of pasta you wish to eat is more like a Frisbee! Dry cereal, before you add milk (remember, also not on the challenge!) should be about the size of a tennis ball too. Bread is one slice and a roll is the size of well, a roll. However, if you make something like banana bread cut it to the size of a normal dinner roll. Which, come to think of it, is about the size of a tennis ball too!

Fruits and Veggies- Yay for fruits and veggies! Fruits, because of their natural sugar content, are only to be eaten once or twice a day. You should eat as many vegetables as you can on the 30-Day Challenge. After the challenge, unless you have an issue with sugar, you should try to get in 4 servings of both fruits and vegetables a day. Okay, so if you are going with fresh fruit you can fall back on the tennis ball rule. If it is dried fruit, then eyeball half a tennis ball! Larger amounts of vegetables can be eaten at once so think softball. A serving of fruit juice or vegetable juice would be 6 ounces.

Remember though if you have a problem with weight or sugar and during this challenge skip the fruit juice and eat the whole fruit only.

Everything else- The last food category is a mix of everything else. This includes your oils, fats, and sweets! NO sweets for thirty days! Remember, if you cheat even one day then you have to start over! Who wants to do that, right? So, when it comes to chocolate or candy think ping pong ball. Salad dressing is also a ping pong ball. That does not seem like a lot but if you are dipping your veggies into the salad dressing then it will last a lot longer! If it is something full of air, think chips or popcorn, it would be about a softball or ½ cup. ½ cup is unfortunately, or fortunately (depending on your disposition) not as much as you think it is. Go look at your measuring cup, you'll see! So, to help you on your challenge journey, on the next page you will find a concise "eyeball" list that you can print out and tape to your fridge or stick in your wallet.

## JUST "EYEBALL" IT

- ❖ Meat-playing cards
- ❖ Nuts or butters- ping pong ball
- ❖ Fruits-tennis ball
- ❖ Veggies-softball
- ❖ Juices- 6 ounces
- ❖ Chocolate, Sweets- ping pong ball
- ❖ Salad Dressing- Ping pong ball
- ❖ Chips, popcorn, pretzels- softball

# HOW TO "HEALTHY UP" YOUR HOME

When you are working through the 30-day whole food challenge or you are making a lifestyle change toward optimal health then you need to make some changes in your kitchen and the rest of your home. They are simple and easy and you will be glad that you took the time to do it.

1. Get rid of everything- That is right. Toss it, donate it, however you want to do it just get the stuff you can't eat out of the house. (I prefer that you donate it!) Now, if there are things your kids eat that you will keep I will go over what to do with that later. Be ruthless as you go through the house. Alcohol is out so wrap up the bottles you have unopened and Voila! You have gifts for the next event you go to. Say good bye to your condiments too, unless you need to keep ketchup and mustard for the kids toss out the rest. Toss out the salad dressings, barbeque sauces and more. Read the labels and if you see anything that does not belong then pitch it.

You cannot make a difference in your life if you do not start with a clean slate.

2. Get a fruit bowl- Take that fruit bowl and display it on the kitchen table and fill it up with apples and oranges. Get a banana hammock and hang up a bunch of ripe bananas. You know the principle "out of sight out of mind"? This is the same thing in reverse. Yes, we are going to use reverse psychology on ourselves! Now our mantra is "in sight, in mouth"! This will work for your kids too, when they come breaking done the door after school starving and can't find any chips or cookies they will grab up that fruit! Keep your prepped food in the fridge in clear Ziploc bags, clear Tupperware and use plastic wrap. You can't eat what you can't see, right? Remember…"IN SIGHT-IN MOUTH"

3. Say Goodbye to the Food Club- Stop shopping in bulk. This only works if you are buying meat to freeze because you can get it on sale or buying bottled water since it lasts forever. Fruits and veggies though do not last

forever so get in the habit of shopping once or twice a week. You will have just the right amount of food in the house and meal prep will be a breeze since you are only doing a week or partial week at a time. Throwing out food is such a waste of money so it is important to buy the right amount of fruits and vegetables that you will eat in that time period and then eat them!

4.  No more meals on the go- I know with a busy life it is hard sometimes to not eat meals on the move. However, I do encourage you to try to do this whenever possible. Not only have studies shown that taking the time to eat at the table helps the diner feel fuller sooner and learn to listen to their bodies "I'm full" cues but also aids in digestion and has the wonderful side effect of bringing the family together for some quality time.

5.  Bye-Bye Couch Snacks- Eating on the couch while watching television or reading a book can lead to mindless snacking. Now, on this diet if you are snacking on something like carrots no big deal, right? But we are trying

to make lifestyle changes here and this is one of them. So, make a new rule in the house. No eating on the couch!

6. Use smaller plates- Using smaller plates is a genius idea. A lot of us are hardwired to finish the food on our plates so when you have a smaller plate you eat less. Also, once you learn portion sizes you may not be feeling up your big plates all the way which can leaving you feeling deprived even though you are not. If you can't buy smaller plates, then simply fill up half of your plate with salad. Heck, do that on the smaller plates too! Salad is filling, has a satisfying crunch and you can eat it all day long.

Follow these tips and you are setting yourself up to succeed. You can do this!

"Courage is the power to let go of the familiar."
~Raymond Lindquist

# Chapter 7- SAMPLE MEAL PLANS

Being organized over the course of this 30-day whole food challenge is extremely important. As we have talked about it is easy to feel overwhelmed on this 30-day challenge and the lure of easy food is always out there. So, what you need to do is plan, prep and then the execution is simple!

Having sample meal plans is a great tool. You can choose to either follow the meal plans exactly or you can simply use them as a stepping stone to create your own weekly lists. The internet is full of whole food recipes and there is no shortage of combinations you can arrange whole foods in to create a delicious and satisfying meal.

## SAMPLE BREAKFAST PLANS

WEEK ONE

Day 1-½ cup of blueberries

2 eggs scrambled with diced tomatoes, salt is okay

Day 2-3 slices bacon (cured in salt, not sugar)

½ cup sliced strawberries with minced fresh mint

Day 3-2 eggs scrambled with sliced mushrooms and onions

Handful of sunflower seeds

Day 4-banana

3 slices bacon (cured in salt, not sugar)

Day 5-20 frozen grapes

2 fried eggs


Day 6-Denver Scramble

Orange


Day 7-Sweet Potato Hash browns

3 slices bacon

WEEK 2-

Day 1-Cinnamon Apples

Scrambled Eggs

Day 2-Scrambled Eggs

Bacon

Day 3-Banana

Denver Scramble

Day 4- cup of blueberries

3 slices bacon

Day 5- Fried egg

Homemade sausage

Day 6- Eggs with salsa

3 slices bacon

Day 7- Fruit Salad

Sweet Potato Hash browns

WEEK 3-

Day 1- ½ cup of grapes and mandarin oranges

      3 slices of bacon- cured with salt not sugar

Day 2- Banana

      Denver Scramble

Day 3- 1 apple

      Omelet with mushrooms and onions

Day 4- ½ cup fresh blueberries

      2 fried eggs

Day 5- 2 pineapple spears

      3 slices bacon


Day 6- 1 peach

      Eggs scrambled with tomato


Day 7- 3 slices of bacon

      Sweet potato hash browns

Week 4-

Day 1- Apples and Cinnamon

      3 slices of bacon

Day 2- Denver Scramble

      Banana

Day 3- Fried Egg

      Sweet  potato hash browns

Day 4- Scrambled eggs with sautéed mushrroms and onion

      3 slices of bacon

Day 5- 2 eggs scrambled with fresh tomato and onion, chopped

      2 pineapple spears


Day 6- Denver Scramble

      Orange


Day 7- 3 slices of bacon

      Sweet potato hash browns


Day 1- Apples and Cinnamon

      3 slices bacon


Day 2- Banana

      Denver Scramble

# Chapter 8- RECIPES FOR BREAKFAST

Your mother probably told you a thousand times that breakfast is the most important meal of the day and she is right! Breakfast is what fuels you for the day and a filling breakfast will keep you going strong until your next meal. When you have a good, healthy breakfast your energy levels will be up and you can avoid that mid-morning "Gotta grab something from the vending machine to stay awake slump". I like to eat my fruit in the morning as well as some protein like eggs or bacon (salt cured-make sure to check the labels and skip the bacon that is sugar cured.)

You will find that making a habit of eating breakfast over the course of the 30-day whole food challenge you are embarking on will be a habit you continue after the month is up. If your kids skip breakfast before school, then do them a favor and get them into the habit as well. Studies show that kids that eat a satisfying healthy breakfast are more alert at school, do better on tests and retain the knowledge easier. It is hard to concentrate and learn on an empty stomach. It is a habit that will benefit the whole family so add it into your morning routine! It only takes a few minutes to eat a banana or scrambled eggs and it will benefit your family immensely.

## SEED CEREAL

You may be thinking, are you serious? Seed cereal? What am I? A bird? I know, I know, it does sound a little weird but it is yummy and it is allowed on this challenge so why not give it a try?

Ingredients-

- ✓ 1 cup chia seeds
- ✓ ½ cup hemp seeds
- ✓ 1 cup ground flaxseed
- ✓ 2 ¼ tsp cinnamon
- ✓ ½ tsp ginger
- ✓ ½ tsp nutmeg

This is your cereal mix. You can store it in a Tupperware container.

Directions-

1. Pour 1/3 cup cereal into a bowl.
2. Mash a medium size banana up and add to the bowl
3. Add 1/3 cup almond milk- may want more or less depending on the consistency you desire.
4. Add 1 tsp of ghee (optional)

5.  Microwave 90 seconds to 2 minutes.

6.  Enjoy!

I hope you like this recipe! My aunt swears by this recipe and even her kids enjoy it! I hope yours do too! It is so easy to make you can even pack some while you are traveling to avoid the temptations of a hotel continental breakfast.

# DENVER SCRAMBLE

Have you heard of a Denver Scramble? It is delicious! Scrambled eggs with ham and peppers, it adds a little Southwest flair to your day!

Ingredients-

- ✓ 3 Eggs
- ✓ Ham- cooked and chopped (1/4 cup)
- ✓ Bell Peppers- you can use red, green, yellow or orange or add all the colors for a beautiful dish! (1 pepper's worth)- chopped
- ✓ Salt
- ✓ Onions- chopped- about ¼ onion

Some people choose to sauté their veggies and some prefer the crispness of the raw veggies. It is completely up to you. This recipe is for one person but is easily doubled, tripled, etc.

Directions-

1. Chop up the veggies you plan to use. Mix them in a bowl with the ham.
2. Get out three eggs. Place in small bowl. Whisk. Mix into the veggie bowl.

3. Scramble egg mixture as you normally would.
4. Add salt to taste!
5. Enjoy!

It is as easy as that and is quite delicious! See, you can enjoy a delicious breakfast without butter and cheese!

# SWEET POTATO HASHBROWNS

Sweet potato hash browns are delicious! You may be like I was before I started this challenge. You think sweet potatoes and your first reaction is eww! But, you will most likely find that you DO like sweet potatoes, just like I did! You can have white potatoes on this diet but sweet potatoes should be used more often.

Ingredients-

- ✓ 2 sweet potatoes- sliced, grated or cubed
- ✓ Green onions-1/4 cup or more- I love onions so I add more
- ✓ 1 tsp. salt- I do prefer sea salt in recipes, so delicious and adds a nice thick salt crystal
- ✓ 1/8-1/4 cup oil- you can use coconut oil or olive oil

Directions-

1. Get out your frying pan
2. Add a little oil and allow it to heat up to a med-high
3. While heating stir together potatoes, onions, and salt

4. When hot, add a little more oil

5. Dump the potato mixture into the frying pan

6. Cook about 10 minutes or until the potatoes are a beautiful golden brown

7. Keep stirring as you cook so the potatoes do not burn or stick to the pan

8. When finished dump the finished product on a paper towel covered plate to soak up any oil

9. Place the hash browns on a new plate with the rest of your breakfast!

10. Enjoy!

# SCRAMBLED EGGS

Scrambled eggs are easy, delicious and good for you! Just in case you do not know how to make scrambled eggs, here are the directions!

Ingredients-

- ✓ 3 eggs
- ✓ Salt

Directions-

1. Warm up your skillet with a splash of olive oil.
2. Break your eggs into a bowl and whisk them.
3. Dump them in skillet constantly stirring and moving about until they are soft and fluffy.
4. Slide onto a plate.
5. Enjoy!

# SCRAMBLED EGGS WITH FRESH TOMATO

I know this is self-explanatory but here goes anyway!

Ingredients-

- ✓ Cooked scrambled eggs
- ✓ 1 tomato- minced

Directions-

1. Chop up your tomato into small pieces.
2. Stir with scrambled eggs.
3. Enjoy!

## SCRAMBLED EGGS WITH SAUTEED MUSHROOMS AND ONIONS

When you get to side dishes you will learn how to sauté mushrooms. To make this sauté the onions with the mushrooms. Just cut the onions into tinier pieces than the mushrooms since they can cook longer.

Ingredients-

- ✓ 1 onion and a cup of mushrooms- sautéed
- ✓ Scrambled eggs

Directions

1. Sauté your onions and mushrooms.
2. Scramble your eggs.
3. Mix together.

# FRUIT AND NUT "PARFAIT"

This is a take on the classic parfait. There is no dairy. Instead you will use nuts, fruit and a sprinkling of cinnamon and cocoa. It is delicious and offers a great boost of protein to start your morning off right.

Ingredients-

- ✓ Handful of almonds
- ✓ Handful of pecans
- ✓ Handful of walnuts
- ✓ Banana
- ✓ Raspberry

Directions-

1. Mix the nuts together.
2. Slice the bananas.
3. Mix the bananas and raspberries together with a sprinkling of cinnamon and cocoa.
4. Layer the fruit and the nuts.
5. Enjoy!

# Chapter 9- RECIPES FOR LUNCH

Lunch is a great time to enjoy a salad. Chicken salad, tuna salad, steak salad, fruit salad, veggie salad, salmon salad and more. Salads can be created using so many different ingredients you can enjoy a different salad every single day!

Add vegetables and fruits of various colors to ensure maximum nutrition and create a pleasing to look at dish. Add something like cabbage or nuts for a satisfying crunch on top.

If you go to lunch and order a salad be sure to ask for vinegar and oil on the side to dress your salad with as their dressings will most likely be processed.

# TUNA SALADS

Tuna salad is a filling choice for lunch on the 30 Day Whole Foods Challenge. You may be used to eating your tuna salad on bread or crackers but it is just as satisfying on its own or wrapped up in a crisp lettuce leave. You can also spread on cucumber slices, carrot sticks, celery sticks, Granny Smith Apples or tomatoes. You will want to start with canned tuna and if you want to season, add your own. There are many flavored tuna pouches on the market today but there is a good chance that they will contain MSG or sugar so it is advisable to avoid them and add your own seasoning. There are many uniquely flavored ways to create tuna salad. The possibilities are endless. Here are my two favorite tuna salad recipes compatible with the whole foods challenge.

1. Avocado Tuna Salad- this recipe used avocado instead of mayonnaise to make a creamy yet delicious tuna salad.

Ingredients-

✓ Can tuna

- ✓ Avocado- generally a half of an avocado works well
- ✓ 2 carrot sticks- chopped small
- ✓ 1 celery stick- chopped small
- ✓ ¼ onion- chopped small
- ✓ 1 tsp lemon or lime juice
- ✓ Seasoning- 1/8 tsp of both chili powder and cumin

Directions-

a. Drain the can of tuna
b. Mash the avocado
c. Mix all ingredients together
d. Eat with a fork or wrap in a crisp lettuce leaf
e. Enjoy!

2. Balsamic Tuna Salad- Balsamic vinegar is a great addition to many meals and adds an intense boost of flavor to any dish. This salad is more like a traditional salad with the addition of tuna.

Ingredients-

- ✓ 1 cup greens- add spinach or kale for an extra health boost!
- ✓ 1 onion-sliced
- ✓ 1 can tuna- drained
- ✓ 1 tomato- sliced
- ✓ Sliced cucumber
- ✓ Balsamic Dressing

Directions-

a. Slice your veggies.
b. Drain your tuna.
c. Layer a plate with the greens.
d. Place veggies on top.
e. Fork tuna across top of plate
f. Drizzle with Balsamic Dressing
g. Enjoy!

Some people like to add olives to this salad since it has a bit of a Mediterranean flair. I don't personally like olives but I know a lot of you do. Green or black will work!

# STEAK SALAD

Steak salad is one of those salads that fills you up and never leaves you feeling deprived. It is delicious and while there is a recipe here for steak salad you can mix and match ingredients as much as you like!

Ingredients-

- ✓ Strips of Steak-sliced thin
- ✓ Mixed Greens
- ✓ ¼- ½ sliced red onion-sliced thin
- ✓ ½ cucumber-sliced thin
- ✓ Balsamic Dressing

Directions-

1. Lay a bed of mixed greens on your plate.
2. Mix onion, cucumber and steak and then cover bed of mixed greens.
3. Drizzle Balsamic Dressing over the salad.
4. Enjoy!

# SWEET POTATO BITES

Sweet Potato Bites are delicious and healthy and the perfect complement to any lunch. They replace French fries and your body will thank you for that! They are simple to make yet delicious!

Ingredients-

- ✓ 3 Sweet Potatoes- cubed or chunked
- ✓ Tablespoon olive oil
- ✓ Italian Seasoning

Directions-

1. Get an 8X8 glass pan or something similar and place potatoes inside after you have chunked them.
2. Pour olive oil over the potatoes
3. Sprinkle with seasoning
4. Stir it all together
5. Bake at 375 for about 45 minutes. Stir at 30 minutes. Potatoes should be soft in the middle and easily cut with a fork.
6. Enjoy!

# Chapter 10- RECIPES FOR MAIN DISHES

Dinner can be the hardest meal of the day to plan for while you are doing the 30-day whole food challenge. You are tired, the whole family is at the table and you just had salad for lunch. So, what to do?

You can make a lot of the same foods you did before and just omit the bread products. Like tacos with no shells, hamburgers with no bun and stir-fry with no rice. (some people make "fried rice" with cauliflower and rave about it). You can even substitute veggies for bread by using a portabella mushroom for a bun and a crisp lettuce leaf for a tortilla.

Meal planning will make it easier and soon enough you will be in the groove.

# CARNE ASADA- NO TORTILLAS ALLOWED

Mexican food is easy to make at home and even though you cannot have the bread portion, like tortillas and taco shells, it will taste just as delicious! If you really want to wrap up your dish in something use a crisp piece of lettuce!

Ingredients

- ✓ 1 lb flank steak, thin
- ✓ 2 TBSP olive oil
- ✓ Lime- fresh lime juice is so yummy!
- ✓ 2 cloves of garlic- minced up
- ✓ ½ tsp salt
- ✓ ¼ tsp pepper
- ✓ ½ tsp chili powder
- ✓ ½ tsp garlic powder
- ✓ ½ tsp cumin
- ✓ ¼ tsp oregano

✓ ½ tsp paprika

Directions-

1. Combine the oil and seasonings with the lime juice and stir.
2. Place the steak in the mixture and allow to marinate for atleast an hour.
3. When you are ready set your oven to broil and make sure the top rack is as high as it can go.
4. Broil the steak for 6 minutes on one side and 6 on the other. If you are like me cook it a little longer. I like mine really well done!
5. Slice the steak up.
6. Add a little guacamole or some fresh onions and tomatos.
7. Enjoy!

# GRILLED CHICKEN

Chicken on the grill is simply delightful! On this diet you cannot use barbeque sauce however you can use your own Italian dressing. It is easy to grill and it is delicious!

Ingredients-

- ✓ Italian Dressing
- ✓ Thin Chicken Breasts

Directions-

1. Marinate the chicken in the dressing overnight.
2. When ready grill the chicken, flipping frequently and basting often, until it is cooked completely through.
3. Enjoy!

This is a great dish to make too much of so you can stick some in the fridge to eat over a salad for the next few days.

# ROASTED CHICKEN AND BROCOLLI

This is not a boring chicken dinner but one that you can bring out for company regardless of whether your guests only eat whole foods. They will still love it!

Ingredients-

- ✓ Head of broccoli
- ✓ Whole chicken, divided into pieces
- ✓ 3 tablespoons olive oil, divided
- ✓ ½ tsp sea salt
- ✓ ½ tsp rosemary

Directions-

1. Preheat your oven to 450 degrees
2. Mix the broccoli with the seal salt, rosemary and 2 tablespoons olive oil
3. Rub oil over the outside of the chicken pieces; coating the skin so it will crisp up.
4. Roast in baking pan covered with foil for 4o minutes.

5. Remove foil and roast under 20 minutes, chicken temperature should reach 170 degrees.
6. Enjoy!

# EASY POT ROAST IN THE CROCKPOT

This has been a favorite recipe in my household since I was a child long before anyone had ever heard of the whole foods craze or 30 day whole food challenge.

Ingredients-

- ✓ 1 beef roast
- ✓ Water
- ✓ Carrots
- ✓ Potatoes
- ✓ Salt
- ✓ Pepper
- ✓ Garlic powder

Directions-

1. Place beef in the crock pot.
2. Cover almost all of the roast with water.
3. Chop up 2 carrots or grab a handful of baby carrots and place in crockpot.
4. Chop up 4 potatoes, I like to use red, and place in crockpot
5. Sprinkle a little salt, pepper and garlic powder.

6. Cook on low for 8 hours.

7. When it is done cooking it should shred easily; if you plan to shred it.

8. Enjoy!

# EASY ROASTED CHICKEN

This is another recipe that I have been eating since I was a child and now serve to my children and granddaughter.

Ingredients-

- ✓ Whole chicken
- ✓ 2 tsp olive oil

Directions-

1. Remove the insides from the chicken cavity.
2. Rinse and pat dry.
3. Rub oil all over the chicken.
4. Roast according to directions on chicken label.
5. Enjoy!

# BEEF AND VEGETABLES STIRFRY

This is a dish that you can change up as much as you want to fit your own needs and it will be delicious each and every time! This is a family-sized meal.

Ingredients-

- ✓ 1 pound ground beef
- ✓ 1 onion
- ✓ 1 head of broccoli
- ✓ 2 TBSP olive oil
- ✓ 2 TBSP mixed garlic

Directions-

1. Chop up the vegetables.
2. Add the oil to a skillet and turn onto medium heat.
3. Cook vegetables for 5-7 minutes.
4. Add ground beef and cook until there is no pink left. Chop as you go so the beef stays fine.
5. Add in the garlic for the last five minutes of cook time.
6. Enjoy!

# Chapter 11- RECIPES FOR DRESSINGS AND MORE TOPPINGS

Store Dressings, marinades and toppings are a no-no. You will need to make these yourself. However, it is not that big of a deal because these things are easy to make and there are thousands of recipes for them on the internet. You could seriously make a 1000 different recipes for dressings and marinades in a row!

# BALSAMIC DRESSING

Balsamic Dressing adds a punch of flavor to any salad. This is a basic recipe for the dressing but as you begin to explore the flavors you like, feel free to change it up!

Ingredients-

- ✓ ½ cup balsamic vinegar- this is basic balsamic vinegar but it does come in other flavors
- ✓ ½ cups olive oil- extra virgin olive oil is suggested for dressings
- ✓ 3 cloves of garlic- diced
- ✓ Salt to taste- add just a sprinkle at a time

Directions-

1. Combine ingredients in a mason jar.
2. Shake profusely.
3. When extra virgin olive oil gets too cold it can get thicker, so let it sit out before using if this happens or run under a little warm water until it is liquid again.

# MAYONNAISE

Mayonnaise is a condiment some people cannot live without! Here is a recipe that you can use to get mayonnaise back into your life but since you are on the 30-day whole food challenge use it sparingly.

- ✓ ½ tsp lime juice
- ✓ 1 tablespoon egg white
- ✓ 1/8 teaspoon dry mustard
- ✓ 1/8 teaspoon sea salt
- ✓ 1 clove garlic-minced
- ✓ 4 tablespoons olive oil, divided

Add in seasonings to get new flavors for different meals.

Directions-

1. Put everything except for 3 tablespoons of olive oil into the food processer and puree the mixture until smooth and creamy.
2. Add in the remaining olive oil a little bit at a time while continuing to mix.
3. Enjoy!

You can keep this in the fridge for 7-10 days. You may need to stir again each time before using.

# GUACAMOLE

Guacamole is delicious and easy to make! It is great to dip veggies in, add to salads and top meat with. You can add different spices and minced veggies in to create new and different variations.

Ingredients-

- ✓ 1 ripe avocado
- ✓ ¼ small red onion-minced
- ✓ 1 tsp cilantro
- ✓ ¼ tsp sea salt or pink sea salt
- ✓ 1 tbsp. lime juice

Directions-

1. Place everything in a bowl and mash it together.
2. Enjoy!

# ITALIAN SALAD DRESSING

Yum! Homemade salad dressing is delicious and so much healthier than the stuff you get in the store.

Ingredients-

- ✓ 6 tablespoons oil- I use extra virgin olive oil or canola
- ✓ 2 tablespoons vinegar- balsamic or red wine work well as does white vinegar
- ✓ 1 tablespoon water
- ✓ ¼ tsp salt
- ✓ ½ tsp Italian Seasoning- no sugar added
- ✓ Half of 1/8 tsp of black pepper

Directions-

1. Mix seasonings together in a jar.
2. Add vinegar.
3. Add water.
4. Shake and chill.
5. Enjoy!

# Chapter 12- RECIPES FOR SIDES

Sides are what every protein needs. They are like your protein's back-up dancers! So, try a different side dish every night and see which ones you like the most and then feel free to experiment with different spices and combinations.

# GREEN BEANS AND BROCCOLI

One of my favorite ways, even before this challenge, was to boil green beans or broccoli and mix them with a little olive oil and garlic salt. It is simply delish and goes wonderful with any dinner!

Ingredients-

- ✓ Green beans or broccoli
- ✓ 2 tbsp. olive oil
- ✓ Garlic salt to taste

Directions-

1. Start water boiling at medium-high heat.
2. When the water is boiling add the vegetables.
3. Boil for 5-7 minutes.
4. Drain.
5. Mix with olive oil and garlic salt.
6. Enjoy!

Depending on how many veggies you make at a time you may need a little more or less olive oil. Basically, you only need enough just to coat the vegetables so the garlic salt will stick to the greens.

# SAUTEED MUSHROOMS

Yum! Yum! Yum! Sautéed mushrooms are oh so delicious! Baby Bella mushrooms are my favorite, I think they have a little more flavor. However, white mushrooms will work just as well. We will sauté the mushrooms in olive oil and garlic salt.

Ingredients-

- ✓ 8 oz. mushrooms
- ✓ 2 tbsp. olive oil
- ✓ Garlic salt to taste

Directions-

1. Heat up your frying pan with a little olive oil.
2. When it is nice and hot dump in the mushrooms.
3. Cook about 5-7 minutes. Some people like their mushrooms a little softer and some people, like me, enjoy them crispier.
4. When the mushrooms are just about done sprinkle them with garlic salt and cook about another minute.
5. Dump on a paper towel covered plate.
6. Enjoy!

# AVOCADO SALAD

Avocado is one of those things that is perfect in a variety of dishes. Some of you may have only seen it in guacamole! However, it is good in salad too! Try this one out today!

Ingredients-

- ✓ 1 ripe avocado, peeled and sliced
- ✓ 2 tomatoes, sliced
- ✓ 1 red onion, peeled and sliced
- ✓ 1 tbsp. olive oil
- ✓ 1 tbsp. lemon or lime juice- your choice!
- ✓ 2 tbsp. fresh cilantro, chopped fine

Directions-

1. Slice all of your veggies and place in a bowl.
2. Stir your oil, juice and cilantro together.
3. Mix the liquid with the veggies.
4. Enjoy!

This salad will taste really good a little chilled so take your veggies right out of the fridge and enjoy immediately!

# TOMATO AND ONION SALAD

This has been one of my favorite dishes since before I even knew what a Whole 30 Challenge was and thankfully it is just as delicious and fits right into the parameters of the challenge. This is a great, clean side dish to any meal.

Ingredients-

- ✓ 2 tomatoes, chunked
- ✓ 1 onion, any kind, peeled and chunked

Directions-

1. Chop up your veggies.
2. Drizzle your favorite dressing on top of them. The balsamic would work quite nicely!
3. Enjoy!

# SIMPLE TOMATO

This is not really a recipe but a tasty and easy way to get in a side dish as well as an extra serving of veggies!

Ingredients-

- ✓ Tomato
- ✓ Sea Salt
- ✓ Balsamic Vinegar

Directions-

1. Slice a tomato- Roma tomatoes are very good for this recipe.
2. Sprinkle the slices with some sea salt.
3. Drizzle with a little balsamic vinegar.
4. Enjoy!

## SAUTEED CAULIFLOWER

This is a delicious side dish and a great way to get your family (or yourself!) eat broccoli.

Ingredients-

- ✓ Green onion- 6-chopped small
- ✓ ½ head of cauliflower
- ✓ 2 tablespoons olive oil
- ✓ 2 tablespoons minced garlic

Directions-

1. Chop the green onion into small pieces.
2. Chop the cauliflower into small pieces.
3. Heat the oil in your skillet.
4. When oil is hot, add in cauliflower, garlic and onion.
5. Sauté 4-6 minutes until cauliflower is golden brown.
6. Enjoy!

# Chapter 13- RECIPES FOR "DESSERTS"

You may not think that the Whole Foods Challenge leaves a lot of room to enjoy dessert and you would be right to a point. Having a sweet treat to cap off the end of the day is a nice boost to your motivation! There are ways that you can incorporate a dessert into the picture without cheating on your challenge. You have a powerful ingredient that you can use. Fruit! You might be surprised what a sprinkling of cinnamon does to liven up a piece of fruit and even convince your kids that "Yes, this is real dessert!" You will know though that what it is simply a healthy snack that happens to be naturally sweet. Just like you!

# FRUIT SALAD

Fruit salad is a nice thing to make on your prep days so you are always able to grab some. Remember though, apples and bananas, while delicious, do not last long after being sliced, so add those right before eating.

Ingredients-

- ✓ Cup of green grapes, rinsed
- ✓ Cup of purple grapes, rinsed
- ✓ Can of mandarin oranges
- ✓ 1 banana added before eating
- ✓ 1 can chunked pineapple

Directions-

1. Rinse and chop your fruit
2. Stir it together
3. Add in banana when you are ready to eat the fruit salad
4. Enjoy!

# APPLES AND CINNAMON

Yum! This is a delicious sweet treat that packs all the nutrients of apples along with a sprinkling of cinnamon to tie it all together. This recipe makes enough for two.

Ingredients-

- ✓ 2 TBSP ghee
- ✓ 2 apples
- ✓ Cinnamon

Directions-

1. Peel the apples.
2. Slice the apples thin.
3. Melt the ghee in a skillet over medium heat.
4. Cook the apples over medium heat until they are tender.
5. Remove from heat.
6. Sprinkle with cinnamon.
7. Enjoy!

# Chapter 14-THE 30 DAYS ARE UP, SO NOW WHAT?

Congratulations! You have reached the end of your 30-day whole food challenge! I imagine you are feeling pretty great about now and I am so proud of you for sticking it out! What do you notice? Is your skin clearer? Have you lost weight? (if you haven't weighed yourself yet then go ahead!)

Do you have more energy and notice a clearer mind? Do your joints feel better? Are you more active?

If you are answering yes to my questions, then I would encourage you to keep the momentum going. Now, that doesn't necessarily mean that you will stay on the whole foods diet and that is all right because simply changing your eating habits and avoiding processed foods will continue to make a noticeable difference in your life. Keep resisting sugar! If you miss bread, then have it a few times a week but do not add it back in as a daily staple.

If you started exercising then keep it up because you will continue to feel better, get stronger and reap the rewards which include living a longer and healthier life. You have done so well this month and it just will keep getting easier until you can no longer remember a time when you weren't exercising and eating healthy foods. Can you imagine?

# THE CASE FOR "COOKING IT YOURSELF"

I am currently working on overhauling my kid's diets on a more permanent basis. They ask frequently for snack cakes and store bought cookies. My new mantra has become this…

"If you want a cookie then you have to bake it yourself!"

Surprisingly, it worked! Not very often does a kid or teen want to stop what they are doing and take the time to bake something fresh from scratch. Once or twice a week someone bakes something and the whole family can enjoy it but no longer are there snack cakes piled up in the pantry.

Even more surprising? The kids grab an apple or grapes or a banana when they want that easy snack. The absence of processed snacks plus their desire to eat something quick and easy is actually filling them up with more fruits and vegetables.

I didn't even have to say no! I simply changed the manner in which the cookies got to the table and the rest unfolded like the pages of a beautiful book. The best part about this is it will work for adults too!

When the only quick snack is a bowl of grapes then you grab the bowl of grapes!

## HOW TO STAY HEALTHY AND ADD A FEW THINGS BACK IN

If you decide to add a few things back into your diet I suggest that you add them in one food at a time. This is because you may be sensitive to a food and if you are this will allow you to figure it out. Food allergies are pretty noticeable but food intolerances are less obvious. You may simply feel bloated from a food or get a headache or acne from one food. If you add the food back in and you notice that you feel kind of icky or start getting migraines, then you know you have an issue with that food and you can cut it from your diet entirely.

Have you noticed that real food tastes better? It is almost as if your taste buds had been covered in sludge and they are finally clear! When you eat healthy and whole food tastes delicious!

Do not go back to your old eating habits. Stick with a healthier diet and add back in something like milk but use it less frequently. Try to avoid processed foods at all costs. Ingest sugars occasionally and the same goes with bread. You do not want to undo all the hard work you have accomplished! Believe me, your body will thank you!

## CHALLENGE COMPLETED!

"If you focus on results, you will never change. If you focus on change, you will get results." ~Jack Dixon

YOU DID IT!